Muscle building for hardgainers

From skinny to muscular for men and women

Second edition

Muscle building for hardgainers

From skinny to muscular for men and women

Second edition

Luc Molenaar

Author and publisher: Luc Molenaar
Cover design: Luc Molenaar, image: iStock, John Shepherd
© Luc Molenaar
Contact: info@fitterisbeter.nl

DISCLAIMER
The contents of this book are not intended to replace professional medical advice, medical diagnosis, or medical treatment. Consult a doctor first if there is a medical condition or disease. The performance to be achieved is the responsibility of the performer. Results may vary from person to person.
The author and publisher are not liable for any damage whatsoever (physical or otherwise) caused by the execution of this program.

Preface

"You'll never really get muscular." 'Look at those thin wrists of yours, they'll break when you try!' These comments and many more have been thrown at me on a regular basis. And indeed, I was very skinny and definitely had thin wrists. And I still do. The problem is that many skinny people actually believe these comments. *You're built that way and you'll never be muscular.* But what if I tell you this is nonsense? All 'bullshit'. Not true. You too can build muscle mass! And while doing so, you will get muscle definition faster because of your physique.

There are many people like you, so-called 'hardgainers'. People who are struggling to gain weight. Consider yourself lucky. In any case, this means that you are less likely to gain too much fat and develop associated diseases and ailments. And look at Frank Zane or, more recently, Jeff Cavaliere. Both are very muscular, and both were once very skinny.

But it doesn't come naturally. You're going to have to work hard for it. Nothing is free in life and neither is this. But if you invest the time and adopt the lifestyle that comes with it, you will definitely see results! This book is written especially for people who want to go for it. Thin, skinny, young or old, who want to build muscle mass. If you aren't skinny and have no lanky arms or legs, then put this book away; you will benefit less from this. Other programs may be better.

So dear hardgainer, get to work and make sure those loose-fitting T-shirts become filled with muscle mass! Follow everything in this book to the letter. **<u>Don't skip a step</u>**! This applies to both the nutritional part and the muscle building program. Everything is equally important. Only then will you see real results!

Read the theory thoroughly before you start. Don't go to your (home) gym without knowing exactly what to do there. Every session counts. Every repetition and movement counts. Every calorie counts. And... every moment of rest counts. Start with chapters 1, 2 and 3 where you set out your goals and learn about the basics of nutrition and muscle growth. This is the foundation for everything you will do next so don't skip this. Then you follow the program of chapter 4 and start working on your new self.

So, let's get started! The first step towards a more muscular body has been taken.

Good luck!

Luc.

Table of contents

1. Setting the baseline and determining your goal

'The road to your goal has only two mistakes: not starting and not fully going for it' – ancient Japanese wisdom.

Before you run to the gym, grab some weights and go crazy, know that this doesn't work. You can't build muscle mass without a good plan for nutrition and exercise. And before putting together a good plan, you will have to take a good look at your current self.

First, we need to know what your starting position is. Or, in other words:

- What is your current physique and muscle mass?
- How much do you eat per day or in a week?
- How long do you sleep at night?

And we mean: the reality. Be honest. Don't be embarrassed, it is what it is.

You will soon weigh and measure yourself and take a baseline picture. Don't make yourself heavier or make yourself look more muscular with filters and the like. And, when it comes to nutrition, be honest about what you eat now. You can only progress when you are honest about yourself. Otherwise, the whole program will be one big disappointment!

Step 1: Take a baseline picture

Go to a large mirror, put on your boxer or bikini (and nothing else) and take a picture of your body. One from the front and one from the side. Don't inhale to make your belly look smaller. Don't hold air in your chest to appear fuller. Just stand relaxed. Done? Great! Keep it somewhere safe and don't look at it anymore for the time being. After the program, look at these pictures again and take new ones in the same way. Look at the differences, you'll be amazed at what you've accomplished!

The reason for doing this is important. You will not notice the slight changes your body makes on a daily basis by doing all the workouts of this program. That one tiny half an inch of extra muscle mass is almost unnoticeable when you see yourself in the mirror every day. But trust me, the growth is there. It's a slow process. But… it's totally worth it.

Step 2: Weigh and measure yourself

Length is usually something that doesn't change quickly so you only have to do this at the beginning of the program. Stand upright with your back against the wall and put your heels against the wall. Draw a light pencil mark or a dot just above your head. Measure your height with a measuring rod. Length is a fairly exact measurement (if you do it right).

Weight is another matter. Your weight may fluctuate throughout the day and week. It may even be so that you become more muscular but still (initially) lighter. That is why you do not have to stand on the scale every day during this program. We are in favor of 'measuring is knowing', but we also know that this can lead to frustration if you have suddenly lost a few pounds while you have worked so hard on building your muscle. So why weigh? Well, we need this value to properly determine your objective and calculate how much you need to eat on a daily basis.

So go to that scale and write down the result. Note: your weight is partly influenced by the contents of your bladder and intestines. A good weighing moment is therefore in the morning when you just get out of bed. But if you can't or don't want to wait, write down the time of weighing and do another weighing moment at the same time to still be able to make a bit of a comparison. Weigh yourself in your underwear so that your clothes (that weigh a few pounds) do not add extra weight to the scale. Done? Good. We now have the ingredients to fill out the TDEE calculator. TDEE, you said?

Step 3: Determining your goal

TDEE stands for Total Daily Energy Expenditure, in other words: all the energy you use in a day. If you know how much energy you use in a day, you also know that if you want to gain weight, you have to eat more than that. If you want to lose weight, you will have to eat less.

What you have just read is the basis of the so-called *energy balance*. The energy balance is an important concept in our program and within the fitness and sports world. It comes down to gaining insight into what you use in energy in a day and what you ingest. If this is in balance, you will not lose weight and you will not gain weight. If you use more energy than you normally need to do your daily routine, you lose weight and vice versa.

So: energy intake – energy consumption = result (surplus, balance, deficit)[1].

You can easily determine your TDEE with a calculator. Go to www.fitterisbeter.nl/calculators (yes, 'fiter' is with one 't') and fill in your details:

1. First, fill in your age, gender, height and weight.
2. Select your activity level: none, light (exercise 1-3 times a week), medium (exercise 3-5 times a week), heavy (exercise more than 5 times a week).
3. Determine your goal (in our case this is 'build muscle');

4. Then the calculator asks for your 'macro split'. This is the desired division into carbohydrates, proteins and fats: the so-called macronutrients, also called 'macros'. Many theories have been made about this, but in practice this distribution works best for muscle building: 50% carbohydrates, 25% proteins and 25% fats.

5. Press the 'calculate' button and your personal nutrition plan is made. You now have an indication of the total number of kcal (calories) that you should eat per day, divided into carbohydrates, proteins and fats. Make a note of this.

Step 4: Determine the baseline

Now we still need to know what you eat per day. Keep track of what you eat every day for a week. Be honest and complete. It is best to use an app on your phone for this, for example the 'Food' app from Virtuagym or the MyfitnessPal app. Install such an app on your phone, create a (free) account and fill in your details (height, weight, goal, and your macro-split as calculated above). The app makes the same calculation for you as the TDEE calculator. Once you've done this, you can start tracking your diet.

Such apps are fairly intuitive. So, to use them you don't need days of training. Just fill in what you eat per meal. And yes, sometimes you will have to weigh your food on the kitchen scale! **People are bad at estimating, so weigh!**

An important note for app-users: some people just are not good at reading labels and make mistakes filling in the macronutrients of certain products. Check if this is done right! Some apps have a 'checked' mark for items in the app. These are ok.

For the first week, just eat as you always did and put this in your app (or write this down). There is no good or bad here. During this week you will gain insight into how much you should eat and which of the three macronutrients you eat too little or too much.

Step 5: Visualize your end goal

You might have done this in your head already. But now this is a formal and important step of the program. It's important that you visualize what you want to look like. Be realistic, as a hardgainer you won't immediately look like Arnold Schwarzenegger (world famous body builder) or Celia Gabbiani (world famous cross fitter). But bigger, more muscular and perhaps a six-pack could be feasible. Find a picture of a body you want to look like and save it. This is what you will strive for. And if you lose motivation at some time during the program, take another look at that photo. The person in the photo probably did everything they could to look like this. It probably wasn't easy, but nothing in life comes easy. Work for it! You can do this.

Step 6: Determine sleep time

How many hours do you sleep now? And be honest. You probably don't sleep enough. To gain muscle mass, good sleep is **extremely** important. Sleep at least seven to eight hours (eight hours is better). Go to bed on time if you have to get up early the next morning!

Why is sleep so important? **Muscles grow at rest**. And sleep restores energy. Even if you have been mentally busy, sleep is important for recovery. And going to the gym when you're tired to do a workout is hardly possible and will result in less muscle growth or no growth at all!

Finally

Now that you've gone through these steps, you're ready to start the journey to your new self. Read the next chapter on nutrition and exercise carefully before you start the fitness schedule. Stick to everything written in the book and you will gain muscle mass. Don't be distracted by so-called influencers, others in the gym or your buddies with well-intentioned advice. Everyone has an opinion about building muscle mass and bodybuilding, and they all think they are right! But often these opinions are unfounded and mere hearsay. **Stick to the program!** This works if you do exactly what it says. Only then will you get results! And that's what counts.

2. Nutrition and supplements

'Tell me what you eat, and I will tell you who you are' –
Jean Anthelme Brillat-Savarin

For hardgainers, nutrition is often the most important ingredient in the mix of elements to become more muscular. Of course, training with weights is important, but without enough fuel you will not gain an ounce of muscle mass!

Nutrients

In the previous chapter we have already discussed the macronutrients and the energy balance. So, you know that your diet is made up of carbohydrates, proteins and fats. In addition to these three, there are *other* nutrients that complete the list. These are:

- water;

- vitamins;

- minerals.

You *must* get enough of all these elements to be able to live a healthy life. And by enough we mean not too much and certainly not too little (in your case)! Macronutrients are the most important to focus on. If you eat a healthy and varied diet, you often get enough fiber, vitamins and minerals. It is not necessary to take additional vitamins and minerals in supplement form. Unless you're vegan or vegetarian (but in that case you probably already knew that). For everyone else, this is not necessary if you eat according to the food pyramid. The food pyramid is based on the principle that you take in the following categories during the day[2,7] :

1. Vegetables and fruits.
2. Whole grains (whole wheat bread, whole wheat pasta).
3. Protein (nuts, beans, fish, chicken, whey).
4. Healthy oils (unsaturated fats).

5. Water.

It goes without saying that what you eat should really contribute to a healthy lifestyle and to muscle growth.

Food that does the opposite should disappear from your diet or be consumed to a very limited extent.

What you should eat or drink in moderation or as little as possible are:

1. Alcohol[3]; These are so-called empty calories and therefore do nothing for you in the context of muscle building. It can even backfire. It has a negative effect on your testosterone levels (you need testosterone to build muscle mass, which is the also case for women), it causes muscle acidification and lack of necessary sugars in your muscles (glycogen).
2. Trans fats[4]; unsaturated fats, often processed in the factory that are found in cookies, puff pastry, potato chips, solid frying fat, coffee creamer, pizzas, etc. Eat this in moderation. It increases the risk of cardiovascular disease.
3. Saturated fats: slightly less bad for you than trans fats, but definitely something to eat in moderation. Examples are 40+ cheese, whole milk, chocolate, etc.

Then, what *should* you eat? For muscle growth, **proteins** are very important. And often we don't consume enough of them. You have already calculated how much protein you need, and after the baseline measurement you also know how far you are from that goal. You'll probably have to increase your protein intake.

There are proteins that are quickly absorbed into your body and proteins that are absorbed slowly. The latter make you feel full for a longer amount of time and that is something that can be very useful for those long afternoons. However, for us hardgainers, whether you take slow of fast proteins does not really matter very much because we need to put on some weight and eat more. However, it *is* advisable not to consume all your proteins at once. You'd better eat them throughout the day. That prevents stomach pains and bloating (and also the continuous stream of smelly farts, which doesn't really make anyone happy).

Some people digest protein better than others. The rule of thumb is to take approximately 20-30 grams of protein per meal.

If you do not get enough protein from your diet, a protein supplement is useful. The most sold is whey protein. This is often sold in powder form. It doesn't really matter what you buy. An expensive brand is no better than a cheap brand. Don't fall for the slogan "the purest whey" or anything like it. It is often only a few grams 'more pure' and that is really not worth the extra costs.

Remember: the fitness world has become big because of marketing.

You will often be tempted to buy things you don't need during this program. Don't fall for it. It's a waste of money. But what I *do* recommend is that you take a flavor because flavorless whey tastes like sweaty socks.

Fats are also important, and of course I do not mean the saturated fats I described before. There are also *healthy* fats. Fats that stimulate muscle growth. These include nuts, avocados and olive oil. But you need less fat in volume than the rest. This is because 1 gram of fat equals 7 kcal, whereas 1 gram of protein is only 4 kcal.

Carbohydrates are energy givers, and you need them to perform. Therefore, a low-carbohydrate diet is really not recommended, especially for muscle growth. In fact, during this program, half of your total diet should consist of carbohydrates! But this does not mean that you should run to the sugar pot and empty it! Here too, you have healthier and less healthy options. Almost everything you eat contains carbohydrates. Healthy carbohydrates are to be found in vegetables, fruit and whole grain products. Think of whole wheat pasta, brown rice, potatoes, whole wheat bread, etc.

Like protein, we can also divide carbohydrates into two categories: fast digestible carbohydrates and slow digestible carbohydrates. Fast carbohydrates, as the name implies, are digested quickly and often also cause the so-called 'sugar dip': they give a lot of energy in the short term, but due to blood sugar fluctuations you suddenly get tired shortly afterwards. And then many people start eating again. Maybe you recognize this yourself: first a chocolate bar and an hour later you eat something else because you feel that your energy has run out. This often happens in the afternoon. Therefore, it is better to eat carbohydrates with a low glycemic value. The glycemic value indicates how quickly a carbohydrate type is digested by the body. The lower, the better. Pasta, fruits and legumes have a low value. Soft drinks, sweets and other similar sweets, have a high value. You can look at the glycemic index of a product here: https://glycemicindex.com.

We've pretty much covered all the nutrients now, except for water. We can be brief about this: drink at least two liters of water during the day. When you work out, you can drink a little more during and after exercise. **Without water, there is no muscle growth**.

Supplements

Let's talk about supplements. We already talked about whey and vitamins, but there are others. In fact, there are many more.

In principle, you do not need supplements.

So I don't need a pre-workout shake? No, don't take it! It's often more junk than it is healthy. There is far too much caffeine in it, often as much as 375mg. "On average, healthy adults can ingest about 400 milligrams (mg) of caffeine per day without any problems. For pregnant and breast-feeding women, the advice is not to take more than 200 mg of caffeine over the day," the Nutrition Center says on their website. In an average pre-workout shake there are about six cups of coffee. Quite a lot to take in at once, right?

Pre-workout shakes can also be dangerous due to potential side effects from consuming harmful or unlisted substances. And the current hype of so-called "Dry scooping" is plain stupid. This is a practice of consuming the powder without mixing it with liquid and can result in choking and other health issues like damage to your teeth due to the high citric acid content.

Some pre-workout ingredients, like stimulants, can raise heart rate and blood pressure, potentially causing cardiovascular problems, especially for individuals with pre-existing heart conditions. And Some pre-workouts can have a diuretic effect, leading to dehydration and electrolyte imbalance, especially when combined with excessive caffeine.

My advice: stay healthy and do not use this.

What you can do is have a cup of coffee in advance (one) and eat some carbohydrates. Then you are well charged to do your workout.

Another supplement that I recommend you stay away from is the so-called *testosterone booster*. They really do little or nothing for you and scientific evidence is lacking. Many of these supplements make exaggerated claims about their ability to boost testosterone and improve various aspects of health, which is not accurate.

By the way, I don't have to tell you that you should **stay away** from real anabolic steroids, right? Weight training will increase your testosterone anyway. You don't need any supplements for this. Not even if you're over forty. You still have enough testosterone left to realize muscle building. **Don't be fooled (or don't be a fool)**. I can write a book about the side effects of testosterone supplements. There have been several deaths in the bodybuilding world of people that used (lot's of) steroids. Again, you don't need this. Be natural. Be healthy.

Be beware of the fitness marketing and sponsored influencers. They play on your insecurity as a skinny person and because you want to grow fast and are dissatisfied with yourself, you fall for these advertisements more quickly.

Trust the process you are in. Eat and drink as you calculated and according to what you have read in this chapter. You'll be fine!

Then, a last remark about eating. As a hardgainer you might need to get used to eating (a lot) more than you did before. Make sure you create a schedule with five to six eating moments per day. I suggest you do something like the following:

1. Breakfast. Make sure this consists of protein and healthy carbs. This needs to be approximately 20% of your total kcal.
2. Morning snack: 10% of your total kcal;
3. Lunch: stay on the health track and eat protein, carbs and fats. Approximately 25% of your daily total kcal;
4. Afternoon snack: 10% of your daily kcal;
5. Dinner: again, eat a healthy dinner, consisting of vegetables, meat or fish, and maybe some rice or potatoes, pasta, etc. This needs to be approximately 30% of your total kcal
6. Evening snack: only protein (casein) with some fruit berries, maybe some carbs as well but don't overdo it. Don't eat this right before bedtime but make sure there are a few hours between this eating moment and when you go to sleep. Otherwise, it might result in digestion problems or heartburn. The evening

snack totals the amount of kcal left for that day. In this example it's 5%.

Don't skip an eating moment! If you are not used to eating a lot, you might want to set an alarm for eating. Yes, that helps!

Take eating very seriously. This is the fuel for your muscle growth!

3. Bodybuilding and fitness

'No person has the right to be an amateur in the matter of physical training. It is a shame for a person to grow old without seeing the beauty and strength of which the body is capable.' – Socrates

Bodybuilding and fitness? Right... Bodybuilding is about building bigger muscles. Bringing your body into proportion. Fitness is about your body being fit. Being athletic. There is, as you understand, an overlap between these two concepts.

Traditionally, in the world of bodybuilding, you won't find many cardio activities like running, rowing, cycling, etc. Fitness, on the other hand, is often filled with cardio and a little muscle building. However, both are necessary. And today, fitness has become the concept that often refers to the entire range of weight training *and* cardio. So basically, fitness is everything you can do in the gym. We're going to focus on weight training. The primary goal here is to gain muscle, that's why you bought this book!

How do muscles grow?

So we want muscle growth. Become bigger and stronger. But how do muscles actually grow?

As said in the previous chapter: your diet is always the most important starting point. But we need to put this fuel into work. We will do this with muscle growth exercises. These stimulate the muscle in such a way that it will grow after the workout (not during!) and the next time you do the same workout, you'll notice that you are able to lift a little more weight or do one or more repetitions more than you could do before. That means you have gained muscle mass. Maybe it's not visible yet, but it's there. You've proved it.

For muscle growth exercises, the following concepts are important:

1. The movement itself is always in a correct form.
2. The range of motion from start to end and back is complete.
3. The speed of the motion is as follows: we want a fast contraction and a slow extraction; also called optimal 'time under tension' of the muscle.
4. Every week, the workload increases. This means either you lift a little more weight (the next pin on the

machine, the next weight of the dumbbells, etc.) of you do a few more repetitions. This we call 'progressive overload'.

Progressive overload is a training principle where you gradually increase the demands placed on your body during exercise to stimulate continued improvement. This involves increasing the weight, repetitions, sets, or intensity of your workouts over time. By consistently challenging your muscles, you get muscle growth, strength gains, and improved fitness. The science behind this is, the more you exhaust your muscles, the faster they grow.

But your body is set up to perform movements as efficiently as possible with a minimum of force. Be aware of this:

Lifting weights is something your body doesn't necessarily like.

You feel uncomfortable, feel aches and pains, sweat and – let's face it – you'd rather be done with it quickly. The latter is the reason that many athletes in the gym often rush exercises. But the trick is this: **learn to feel comfortable when you're uncomfortable**. Get used to the annoying feeling of lifting weights; get the most out of it. Only then will your muscles grow. Every time you put in a little more effort. And you *will* be able to do that, but your body might protest from time to time and that's fine.

During the exercises, small tears occur in your muscle tissue. These muscle tears need to be repaired after training. **This happens while you are resting**. Your body transports the necessary nutrition to your muscles, and these will grow so that they are prepared for the next power explosion. If you do this often enough, and increase the intensity regularly, your muscles will grow.

This whole phenomenon is called **'hypertrophy'**. To achieve hypertrophy, a considerable stimulus of the muscle is therefore necessary.

Factors that influence hypertrophy:

1. Training intensity and volume: Lifting heavier weights with fewer repetitions or lighter weights with more repetitions can both induce hypertrophy.

2. Nutrition: Consuming enough protein is crucial for muscle growth and repair.

3. Rest and recovery: Adequate rest allows muscles to repair and rebuild.

4. Genetics: Individual genetic factors can influence how easily someone can build muscle. Hardgainers might not have genetics that easily build muscle, but we'll cover that later when we discuss the types of muscle fiber.

This program is based on hypertrophy. That is why you should always write down how many repetitions you have done and the weight you used, so that you can increase the weight or the number of repetitions after, for example, a week. Always do a little more. And don't overdo it, do it in small steps. Just pick up the next weight on the dumbbell rack or put the pin of the power machine in the next weight. Don't skip weights. And is the next weight too heavy for you? Then first add one or two repetitions per set. Then after a week or two, see if you can use a higher weight. **Using too heavy weights too fast leads to injuries and poor form.**

Super Compensation

If you understand this process and carry it out in your training schedule, it is then important to get enough rest between the exercises of the same muscle group. So, if you train your chest muscles on Monday, you don't immediately train your chest muscles again the next day. There must be a period in between for rest and growth. This phenomenon is also called **'super compensation'**.

The optimal time to train the same muscle group again is somewhere between 48 and 72 hours, according to Leiden University[5]

Now the time between 48 and 72 hours is rather large. How do you know what is optimal for you? Well, that's hard to predict. Everybody reacts differently. If you start with the same muscle group too soon, muscle growth will <u>not</u> occur. So less than 48 hours is definitely not recommended.

Now it is ok to do a few(!) push-ups the next day after a chest session but the intensity should not be high. The program in this book takes into account supercompensation. If you ever develop a schedule yourself, implement enough recovery time between exercises of the same muscle group. Often, training a muscle group twice a week is sufficient (doing it only once is not enough). If, for instance, you plan a chest training on Monday, it is okay to do the same training again on Thursday (or Friday). This way you have enough rest between workouts and your muscles get the chance to grow.

Muscle fibers

For you as a hardgainer, some additional rules apply. For example, you should know that the muscles that are distributed throughout your body can be divided into 'fast twitch' and 'slow twitch' fibers[6]. Fast twitch are also called white muscle fibers. Muscle fibers that can deliver a lot of strength very quickly but cannot sustain this for a very long time. Slow twitch muscle fibers are red (or pink) in color and can provide energy for a very long time. They are smaller (more compact) than the fast twitch muscle fibers, but certainly not unimportant!

You are born with both types. Thank goodness. Genetics determines the exact distribution of muscle fibers. You can't change this. Regularly, slim people are blessed with more slow twitch muscle fibers, but this does not always have to be the case.

The fact is that hardgainers are thin sinewy people with a lot of slow twitch muscle fibers and bodybuilders often possess more fast twitch fibers.

As said, slow twitch fibers are designed for endurance activities. They contract slowly and rely on aerobic metabolism (using oxygen) for energy production, making them resistant to fatigue and ideal for sustained activities like long-distance running or maintaining posture. They tend not to grow in size much, but they do use a lot of energy, also in rest. That's why hardgainers (that possess a lot of these types of fibers) are thin people: the large amount of slow twitch fiber uses lots of energy from the daily food intake not resulting in a surplus of calories that are stored as adipose tissue.

We want to focus on your fast twitch muscle fibers because they grow more and faster in size than slow twitch muscle fibers. And this is primarily done through weight training. And even though you probably have less fast twitch fiber than the average person, it is possible to increase the size of these fibers considerably with the right training. And, because you are a hardgainer, growth is probably more noticeable because you are very slim. If you had a lot of adipose tissue, you would not be able to notice muscle growth at all visually.

Can you convert slow twitch muscle fibers into fast twitch? According to many studies, this is <u>not</u> possible. But research is still taking place, so who knows. Don't focus on that. Focus on the fast twitch muscles; we need to activate them and let them grow. This means that we do not have any endurance sports built into our program. Not even cardio (treadmill, exercise bike, etc.).

What you should know is that muscle growth for you probably does not happen in the same way as with an Arnold Schwarzenegger type. You just don't have that physical ability. But don't worry, you will become bigger and stronger!

Realism in muscle growth

The reason we talk about muscle fibers and growth is to paint a realistic picture. You will definitely become muscular. You will definitely get muscle definition. But you won't become as big as a professional bodybuilder. If this is your goal, it will take years and years. But Frank Zane has also succeeded, so even then there is hope.

But our advice is: focus on what is feasible without having to make very large sacrifices. And do this in a healthy way, without steroids and other junk.

To properly activate fast twitch muscles, explosive exercises are needed[6]. This means that if you pick up a weight, you lift it up (explosive) in 1 second and then lower it again in 2 to 3 seconds (optimal time under tension). This, according to many experts, is the way to grow muscle. After each set (series of repetitions) pause for about 45-60 seconds so that your muscles can fill up again with the fuels used up during the set.

As a hardgainer you have a few disadvantages that we tackle in our program. First of all, you're probably blessed with thinner joints. This means that if you suddenly start lifting heavy weights, you can quickly get injured. **Hence slowly building up weights and always starting with a good warm up is key**.

Furthermore, your entire core (abdominal and lower back muscles) is probably less developed or fragile, so that if you were to lift heavily, you quickly become unstable and can develop back injuries. That's why we have a lot of core workouts in the program. Only when you have developed enough abdominal and back muscle can you start lifting heavier weights.

With this knowledge in mind, you can start the muscle building program. Be alert to aches and pains but try to give everything while training.

Get used to the uncomfortableness of training and 'push yourself'. You can do it.

What has been mentioned in this chapter is only a summary. You don't need more knowledge to achieve your goal. But do you still want to read more about hypertrophy, muscle growth or how muscle fibers work exactly? Then go to: https://www.uc.edu/content/dam/uc/ce/images/OLLI/Page20Content/Muscular20System20s.pdf.

5. Muscle building program step by step

This chapter covers wat you have been waiting for: the program for the next three months and more. Every month your schedule changes slightly, but the basis remains the same.

Consistency is important in muscle growth.

If someone says, 'you need to scare your muscles and do something different every time', ignore that. That's 'bro-science', the so-called science of people in the gym that were always muscular and have no idea what it is like to be a hardgainer! You don't have time for such nonsense. Your goal is clear. And this is the schedule with which you will achieve your goal. That is, if you really go for it, put in the work *and* actually eat what you need to eat. Now, let's get started!

Before you begin

Various exercises are mentioned in this chapter. These exercises are not described in detail in this book. Otherwise, it would be a very, very thick book. All exercises can be found on YouTube (look up Jeff Cavaliere) or exercise books. A tip is to do a few things before you start:

- Learn the exercises and terminology.
- Determine your 1 rep max (1RM); this is the maximum weight you can lift with 1 repetition (two repetitions would not be possible); you can calculate this on www.fitterisbeter.nl/calculators (yes, 'Beter' is with one 't');
- Download a fitness tracker like Virtuagym or MyfitnessPal to track your results; this can of course also be done on paper, but **make sure to always keep track of your results**!

Furthermore, we talk about sets and reps, but what does this mean? A set is a series of repetitions (reps). For example: 3 sets of 12 reps each. This means that you perform three times twelve repetitions (i.e. repetition, rep) of the exercises. Often there is a short break of one minute between sets.

The last concept we need to cover before you start is 'failure'. You will often have to train to failure. This means that you perform a repetition until you can no longer perform the exercise correctly i.e.(right form, right timing).

At home or in the gym?

Do you work out in the gym? Fine, then you're just going to do exactly what the schedule tells you. My tip is: go at a quiet moment if possible or go to an exclusive gym. Then you will have less waiting times at the machines or materials you need. At exclusive gyms everything is often neat, hygienic and there are expert staff who can help you if you have forgotten to do exercise correctly.

Another tip is: read what's on the machine. Every machine is different and there are many brands. Often there is an instruction on a machine that applies to that machine.

If you exercise at home, you will have to purchase some materials. In any case, you will need:
- Adjustable dumbbells (Bowflex, Tunturi, etc.) up to a minimum of 25 kg / 55 lbs per dumbbell.
- Resistance bands with handles and a door anchor.
- Fitness bench and fitness mat.
- Pull-up bar for your door frame.

-    (possibly) Barbell with weights up to about 100 kg /
     220 lbs including the barbell.

Now, let's go to the program!

Week 1

All sets: tighten your muscle for 1 second, lower the weight for 2 to 3 seconds! Rest for 45-60 seconds between sets and 3 minutes after each exercise.

Day	Muscle Group and Exercise	Sets and reps
Monday	Warm up: - 10 push-ups - 10 air squats - 5 chin-ups	
	Chest: - Bench press	2 sets, 12 reps at 70% 1RM
	Back: - Lat pull down (or at home with resistance bands)	2 sets, 12 reps at 70% 1RM

	Chest: - Chest Fly	2 sets, 15 reps at 50% 1RM
	Back: - Back cable row (or at home with resistance bands)	2 sets of 12 at 70% 1RM
	Shoulders: - Shoulder press sitting (dumbbells)	2 sets of 12 reps at 70% 1RM
	Shoulders/back: - Face pulls	2 sets of 15 reps at 70% 1RM, hold 5 seconds after last rep
	Core:	

	- Sit-ups	3 sets of 15
	- Leg raises	3 sets of 15
	Arms:	
	- Bicep curl standing	2 sets of 15 at 70% 1RM
	- Tricep extension pully (or with resistance bands)	2 sets of 15 at 70% 1RM
Tuesday	REST	
Wednesday	Warm up: - 20 sit-ups - 30 air squats	
	Legs: - Leg press machine (or at home: Globlet Squats)	2 sets, 12 reps at 70% 1RM
	Legs: - Hamstring curl machine (or at home with	2 sets, 12 reps at 70% 1RM

	resistance bands)	
	Legs:	
	- Wall sit	120 seconds
	Calves:	
	- Calf raises dumbbells	2 sets, 15 reps at 70% 1RM
	Core:	
	- Crunches	25
	- Flutter kicks	40 (1 rep is 2 legs!)
Thursday	Same as Monday	
Friday	REST	
Saturday	Same as Wednesday	
Sunday	REST	

Week 2

Now do all the exercises a notch heavier. So, grab the next weight. For exercises without weight: do a few more repetitions. Write down your results! All sets: tighten your muscle for 1 second, lower the weight for 2 to 3 seconds! Rest for 45-60 seconds between sets and 3 minutes after each exercise.

Day	Muscle Group and Exercise	Sets and reps
Monday	Warm up: - 10 burpees with push-up - 5 chin ups	
	Chest: - Bench press	2 sets, 12 reps
	Back: - Lat pull down (or at home with resistance bands)	2 sets, 12 reps

	Chest:	
	- Chest Fly	2 sets, 15 reps
	Back:	
	- Back cable row (or at home with resistance bands)	2 sets of 12
	Shoulders:	
	- Shoulder press sitting (dumbbells)	2 sets of 12 reps
	Shoulders/back:	
	- Face pulls	2 sets of 15 reps on, hold 5 seconds after last rep
	Core:	
	- Sit-ups	3 sets of 15
	- Leg raises	3 sets of 15
	Arms:	
	- Bicep curl standing	2 sets of 15

		2 sets of 15
	- Tricep extension pully (or with resistance bands)	
Tuesday	REST	
Wednesday	Warm up: - 20 sit-ups - 30 air squats	
	Legs: - Leg press machine (or at home: Globlet Squats)	2 sets, 12 reps
	Legs: - Hamstring curl machine (or at home with resistance bands)	2 sets, 12 reps

	Legs:	
	- Wall sit	120 seconds
	Calves:	
	- Calf raises dumbbells	2 sets, 15 reps
	Core:	
	- Crunches	25
	- Flutter kicks	40 (1 rep is 2 legs!)
Thursday	Same as Monday	
Friday	REST	
Saturday	Same as Wednesday	
Sunday	REST	

Week 3

Now take all the exercises up a notch. So take the next higher weight again. For the exercises without weight: do a few more repetitions. Write down your results! All sets: tighten your muscle for 1 second, lower the weight for 2 to 3 seconds! Rest for 45-60 seconds between sets and 3 minutes after each exercise.

Day	Muscle Group and Exercise	Sets and reps
Monday	Warm up: - 5 chin-ups - 15 push-ups - 15 sit-ups	
	Chest: - Bench press	2 sets, 12 reps
	Back: - Lat pull down (or at home with	2 sets, 12 reps

	resistance bands)	
	Chest:	
	- Chest Fly	2 sets, 15 reps
	Back:	
	- Back cable row (or at home with resistance bands)	2 sets of 12
	Shoulders:	
	- Shoulder press, sitting (dumbbells)	2 sets of 12 reps
	Shoulders/back:	
	- Facepulls	2 sets of 15 reps on, hold 5 seconds after last rep
	Core:	
	- Sit-ups	3 sets of 15
	- Leg raises	3 sets of 15

	Arms: - Bicep curl standing - Tricep extension pully (or with resistance bands)	2 sets of 15 2 sets of 15
Tuesday	REST	
Wednesday	Warm up: - 20 sit-ups - 30 air squats	
	Legs: - Leg press machine (or at home: Globlet Squats)	2 sets, 12 reps
	Legs:	2 sets, 12 reps

	- Hamstring curl machine (or at home with resistance bands)	
	Legs: - Wall sit	120 seconds
	Calves: - Calf raises dumbbells	2 sets, 15 reps
	Core: - Crunches - Flutter kicks	25 40 (1 rep is 2 legs!)
Thursday	Same as Monday	
Friday	REST	
Saturday	Same as Wednesday	
Sunday	REST	

Week 4

This is the last week of this basic schedule. And again, you take everything up a notch. So, take the next higher weight again. And also, for the exercises without weight: do a few more repetitions. Write down your results! All sets: tighten your muscle for 1 second, lower the weight for 2 to 3 seconds! Rest for 45-60 seconds between sets and 3 minutes after each exercise.

If you were not able to do the exercise with more weight, just write down how far you've come. If you get below 10 reps, drop weight again. Then you weren't ready for an increase. In that case try to raise the weight again a week later.

Day	Muscle Group and Exercise	Sets and reps
Monday	Warm up: - 5 minutes of rowing (or 10 chin-ups) - 10 push-ups - 15 sit-ups	

	Chest:	
	- Bench press	2 sets, 12 reps
	Back: - Lat pull down (or at home with resistance bands)	2 sets, 12 reps
	Chest: - Chest Fly	2 sets, 15 reps
	Back: - Back cable row (or at home with resistance bands)	2 sets of 12
	Shoulders: - Shoulder press, sitting (dumbbells)	2 sets of 12 reps

	Shoulders/back:	
	- Facepulls	2 sets of 15 reps on, hold 5 seconds after last rep
	Core:	
	- Sit-ups - Leg raises	3 sets of 15 3 sets of 15
	Arms:	
	- Bicep curl standing	2 sets of 15
	- Tricep extension pully (or with resistance bands)	2 sets of 15
Tuesday	REST	
Wednesday	Warm up: - 20 sit-ups - 30 air squats	

	Legs:	
	- Leg press machine (or at home: Globlet Squats)	2 sets, 12 reps
	Legs:	
	- Hamstring curl machine (or at home with resistance bands)	2 sets, 12 reps
	Legs:	
	- Wall sit	120 seconds
	Calves:	
	- Calf raises dumbbells	2 sets, 15 reps
	Core:	
	- Crunches	25
	- Flutter kicks	40 (1 rep is 2 legs!)
Thursday	Same as Monday	

Friday	REST	
Saturday	Same as Wednesday	
Sunday	REST	

Intermediate measurement and recalibration of nutrition

After these four weeks, it's time to adjust your feeding schedule. You now train four times a week and you can indicate this in the calculator or your fitness app. In most cases, this means that you have to eat (even) more. **Make the adjustment and eat more**.

Week 5

All sets: tighten your muscle for 1 second, lower the weight for 2 to 3 seconds! Rest for 45-60 seconds between sets and 3 minutes after each exercise. We're adding a set now, to a lot of the exercises. If you don't make it to 12 reps, write down how far you've come.

Day	Muscle Group and Exercise	Sets and reps

Monday	Warm up: - 5 minutes of rowing (or 10 chin-ups) - 10 push-ups - 15 sit-ups	
	Chest: - Bench press	3 sets, 12 reps
	Back: - Lat pull down (or at home with resistance bands)	3 sets, 12 reps
	Chest: - Chest Fly	3 sets, 15 reps
	Back: - Back cable row (or at home with resistance bands)	3 sets of 12
	Shoulders:	

	- Shoulder press, sitting (dumbbells)	3 sets of 12 reps
	Shoulders/back: - Face pulls	2 sets of 15 reps on, hold 5 seconds after last rep
	Core: - Sit-ups - Leg raises	3 sets of 15 3 sets of 15
	Arms: - Bicep curl standing - Tricep extension pully (or with resistance bands)	3 sets of 15 3 sets of 15
Tuesday	REST	
Wednesday	Warm up: - 20 sit-ups - 30 air squats	

	Legs:	3 sets, 12 reps
	- Leg press machine (or at home: Globlet Squats)	
	Legs:	3 sets, 12 reps
	- Hamstring curl machine (or at home with resistance bands)	
	Legs:	120 seconds
	- Wall sit	
	Calves:	3 sets, 15 reps
	- Calf raises dumbbells	
	Core:	
	- Crunches	25
	- Flutter kicks	40 (1 rep is 2 legs!)

Thursday	Same as Monday	
Friday	REST	
Saturday	Same as Wednesday	
Sunday	REST	

Week 6

All sets: tighten your muscle for 1 second, lower the weight for 2 to 3 seconds! Rest for 45-60 seconds between sets and 3 minutes after each exercise.

Day	Muscle Group and Exercise	Sets and reps
Monday	Warm up: - 20 burpees (with push-ups) - 15 sit-ups - 10 chin-ups	
	Chest: - Bench press	3 sets, 12 reps
	Back: - Lat pull down (or at home with resistance bands)	3 sets, 12 reps
	Chest: - Chest Fly	3 sets, 15 reps

	Back: - Back cable row (or at home with resistance bands)	3 sets of 12
	Shoulders: - Shoulder press, sitting (dumbbells)	3 sets of 12 reps
	Shoulders/back: - Face pulls	2 sets of 15 reps on, hold 5 seconds after last rep
	Core: - Sit-ups - Leg raises	3 sets of 15 3 sets of 15
	Arms:	

	- Bicep curl standing	3 sets of 15
	- Tricep extension pully (or with resistance bands)	3 sets of 15
Tuesday	REST	
Wednesday	Warm up: - 20 sit-ups - 30 air squats	
	Legs: - Leg press machine (or at home: Globlet Squats)	3 sets, 12 reps
	Legs: - Hamstring curl machine (or at home with	3 sets, 12 reps

	resistance bands)	
	Legs: - Wall sit	120 seconds
	Calves: - Calf raises dumbbells	3 sets, 15 reps
	Core: - Crunches - Flutter kicks	25 40 (1 rep is 2 legs!)
Thursday	Same as Monday	
Friday	REST	
Saturday	Same as Wednesday	
Sunday	REST	

Week 7

All sets: tighten your muscle for 1 second, lower the weight for 2 to 3 seconds! Rest for 45-60 seconds between sets and 3 minutes after each exercise.

Day	Muscle Group and Exercise	Sets and reps
Monday	Warm up: - 15 sit-ups - 10 chin-ups - 15 push-ups	
	Chest: - Bench press	3 sets, 12 reps
	Back: - Lat pull down (or at home with resistance bands)	3 sets, 12 reps
	Chest: - Chest Fly	3 sets, 15 reps

	Back:	
	- Back cable row (or at home with resistance bands)	3 sets of 12
	Shoulders:	
	- Shoulder press, sitting (dumbbells)	3 sets of 12 reps
	Shoulders/back:	
	- Face pulls	2 sets of 15 reps on, hold 5 seconds after last rep
	Core:	
	- Sit-ups	3 sets of 15
	- Leg raises	3 sets of 15
	Arms:	
	- Bicep curl standing	3 sets of 15
	- Tricep extension pully (or with	3 sets of 15

	resistance bands)	
Tuesday	REST	
Wednesday	Warm up: - 20 sit-ups - 30 air squats	
	Legs: - Leg press machine (or at home: Globlet Squats)	3 sets, 12 reps
	Legs: - Hamstring curl machine (or at home with resistance bands)	3 sets, 12 reps
	Legs: - Wall sit	120 seconds
	Calves: - Calf raises dumbbells	3 sets, 15 reps

	Core:	
	- Crunches	25
	- Flutter kicks	40 (1 rep is 2 legs!)
Thursday	Same as Monday	
Friday	REST	
Saturday	Same as Wednesday	
Sunday	REST	

Week 8

All sets: tighten your muscle for 1 second, lower the weight for 2 to 3 seconds! Rest for 45-60 seconds between sets and 3 minutes after each exercise.

Day	Muscle Group and Exercise	Sets and reps
Monday	Warm up: - 10 chin-ups - 15 push-ups - 15 sit-ups	
	Chest: - Bench press	3 sets, 12 reps
	Back: - Lat pull down (or at home with resistance bands)	3 sets, 12 reps
	Chest: - Chest Fly	3 sets, 15 reps

	Back:	
	- Back cable row (or at home with resistance bands)	3 sets of 12
	Shoulders:	
	- Shoulder press sitting (dumbbells)	3 sets of 12 reps
	Shoulders/back:	
	- Facepulls	2 sets of 15 reps on, hold 5 seconds after last rep
	Core:	
	- Sit-ups	3 sets of 15
	- Leg raises	3 sets of 15
	Arms:	
	- Bicep curl standing	3 sets of 15
	- Tricep extension pully (or with	3 sets of 15

	resistance bands)	
Tuesday	REST	
Wednesday	Warm up: - 20 sit-ups - 30 air squats	
	Legs: - Leg press machine (or at home: Globlet Squats)	3 sets, 12 reps
	Legs: - Hamstring curl machine (or at home with resistance bands)	3 sets, 12 reps
	Legs: - Wall sit	120 seconds
	Calves: - Calf raises dumbbells	3 sets, 15 reps

Day	Exercise	Reps
	Core: - Crunches - Flutter kicks	 25 40 (1 rep is 2 legs!)
Thursday	Same as Monday	
Friday	REST	
Saturday	Same as Wednesday	
Sunday	REST	

After week 8

So, you've completed the first two months! The schedule may have been a bit boring, but it did ensure solid training of your large muscle groups, core, your calves, arms and abs. Maybe you've had muscle pain. That's not a problem; it's part of the game.

Maybe you've had some motivational issues. That happens too. When this happens, think about your goal and trust the process! These bumps make you mentally stronger.

Perseverance is an important ingredient in becoming more muscular.

But now that you've come here, I know you're not a dropout. And
that's great! So let's go to the third month. We're going to train harder again!

Week 9 to 12: bigger muscles coming up!

The last phase of the program: creating superior muscle growth! We are changing the program a bit by again only doing 2 sets per exercise. However, the way we do it is totally different:

1. *The first set: do this until failure with the weight you ended with the last time you did the exercise. This maybe 10, 12 or even 15 reps, doesn't matter. Stop when you feel the muscle is losing energy and you cannot lift the weight anymore (or you can but you will lose form, range-of-motion and time-under-tension).*
2. *Then wait 30-40 seconds*
3. *Then start the second set and do 20 reps with the same weight. Rest as little as possible in between. Stop until you hit 20.*
4. *If you can do the 20 without rest, increase the weight.*
5. *Rest 3 minutes between different exercises.*

For core exercises we will use a slightly different routine as shown in the table below.

Day	Muscle Group and Exercise	Sets and reps
Monday	Warm up: - 10 chin-ups - 15 push-ups - 15 sit-ups	
	Chest: - Bench press	Set 1 to failure, set 2: 20 reps
	Back: - Lat pull down (or at home with resistance bands)	Set 1 to failure, set 2: 20 reps
	Chest: - Chest Fly	Set 1 to failure, set 2: 20 reps
	Back: - Back cable row (or at home with	

	resistance bands)	Set 1 to failure, set 2: 20 reps
	Shoulders: - Lateral raises	Set 1 to failure, set 2: 20 reps
	Shoulders/back: - Face pulls	Set 1 to failure, set 2: 20 reps
	Core: - Sit-ups - Leg raises	50 reps, rest as little as possible in between
	Arms: - Bicep curl standing - Hammer curl stand	For all exercises: Set 1 to failure, set 2: 20 reps

	- Tricep extension pully (or with resistance bands) - Skull crushers	
Tuesday	RUST	
Wednesday	Warming up: - 20 sit-ups - 30 air squats	
	Legs: - Back Squat Smith Machine of Globlet Squats	Set 1 to failure, set 2: 20 reps
	Legs: - Hamstring curl machine (or at home with resistance bands)	Set 1 to failure, set 2: 20 reps
	Legs: - Leg extension	Set 1 to failure, set 2: 20 reps

	Calves: - Calf raises dumbbells	Set 1 to failure, set 2: 20 reps

	Core:
	  - Sit-ups
	  - Shelf
		Until failure
		120 seconds

	Lower back: - Back extension (machine of mat)	Set 1 to failure, set 2: 20 reps
Thursday	Same as Monday	
Friday	REST	
Saturday	Same as Wednesday	
Sunday	REST	

After week 12

Fantastic! You have completed 12 weeks of training! You have trained every muscle group. You have certainly gained muscle mass, and it might show in the mirror! Take that old photo from the beginning out of your desk drawer and compare it to a new photo. Do you see a difference? You have definitely become stronger because you are lifting much more weight than when you started. If you don't see much difference, don't be discouraged. Trust the process. Most hardgainers take a year or more to punt on pounds of muscle.

Never stop!

You are now also familiar with the fitness equipment and exercises and that makes you a more experienced bodybuilder! Now it is important that you continue this. And again, we crack it up a notch.

But first we have to look at your diet. Do you still eat enough? Weigh yourself. Haven't you gained any weight in the past three months? Then you probably need to eat more! Bear in mind: without sufficient nutrition (including water!) there is no muscle growth! Also make sure you have enough rest days between the workouts and sleep 7-8 hours a night.

The schedule you have executed is a so-called 'upper-lower scheme'. This allows you to train all your muscle groups twice a week, which according to many trainers and coaches, is optimal. Training more often than that leads to **overtraining** and less training gives too little growth stimuli.

There are several other 'splits' to be found, but I don't recommend most of them. For example, don't do a so-called 'bro-split'. This cuts your program in such a way that you train each muscle group on one day in the week (i.e chest on Monday, back on Tuesday, etc.) <u>For you, this is not sufficient</u>. I recommend that you either continue with the schedule you are doing now (the schedule of the last four weeks) and after two months do a so-called 'deload week'. This is a week of rest, or a week of quiet training. After that, you can hit it hard again.

In any case, stick to a similar setup as this:
- Monday: Upper
- Tuesday: Rest
- Wednesday: Lower
- Thursday Upper
- Friday: Rest
- Saturday: Lower
- Sunday Rest.

A push-pull scheme can be a good alternative if you are fed up with the above. This may look like this:

Day	Muscle group	Examples
Monday	Chest (Push)	Chest press, incline and flat
	Shoulders (Push)	Arnold press
		Squat
	Leg Press of Squat (Push)	
	Triceps (Push)	Tricep extensions or dips
Tuesday	Rust	
Wednesday	Back (Pull)	Pull-ups
	Leg curls (Pull)	Hamstring curls
	Bicep (Pull)	Bicep curls, preacher curls
Thursday	Rust	
Friday	Push	
Saturday	Rust	
Sunday	Pull	

6. Growing towards your goal

Now that you have worked so hard and long on your new physique, you naturally want to maintain your results or even grow more! Often it takes a year or more before you really start looking like your goal-picture. **Muscle growth takes time**. An inch of arm growth can take a year or two. Fortunately, when you start, you have a kind of 'beginner growth luck'. This means that when you start bodybuilding, your muscles get such a boost that you grow faster for a short time. But this advantage will disappear over time. That is why you will have to train harder and harder each workout to achieve muscle growth. But if you can lift more every time you hit the gym, you are becoming stronger. And that's what you ultimately wanted.

Substitution exercises

Continue to train and be consistent, is the credo here. Stick with your schedule. But adjust something in that schedule every three months, for example change the exercise you do. You can just keep doing an upper-lower schedule but find a substitute for some exercises. There are many ways to train your chest muscles. You can replace a dumbbell press with a barbell bench press or vice versa. This gives your muscle group another stimulus. You can try a vertical chest press machine or indulge in push-ups. These are all exercises for your chest muscles. You can also perform a chest fly on a machine, with cables or lying on a bench with dumbbells. It's all the same movement, but it can just give a new stimulus.

The same goes for all other muscle groups. Pull-ups and the lat-pull-down are similar exercises. A leg press and a squat too. Alternate them once every three months (without changing your schedule per se). Then it gets a bit more exciting because it also has to be fun, right?

Here is a table of exercises you can substitute per muscle group. There are tons of different exercises that 'do the same thing', but this table gives you an idea. If you move further down the bodybuilding road you might find more differentiation per muscle group. For example, your back muscles consist of the trapezius, the latissimus dorsi (i.e. the lats), etc. Each muscle group has its own exercise that stimulates that particular muscle the most, but also targets the surrounding muscle as well. The lat-pull down or pull up targers the latissimus dorsi, but also targets the biceps and other back muscles.

Muscle Group	Barbell	Dumbbell	Machine/Cable	Bodyweight/Band
Chest	Barbell Bench Press	Dumbbell Bench Press	Pec Deck / Cable Crossover	Push-ups / Band Chest Press
Back	Barbell Bent-Over Row	One-Arm Dumbbell Row	Lat Pulldown / Seated Row	Pull-ups / Band Rows
Shoulders	Barbell Overhead Press	Seated Dumbbell Press	Machine Shoulder Press / Cable Lateral Raise	Pike Push-up / Band Shoulder Press
Biceps	Barbell Curl	Alternating Dumbbell Curl	Cable Curl / Preacher Curl Machine	Resistance Band Curl
Triceps	Close-Grip Bench Press	Dumbbell Overhead Triceps Extension	Triceps Pushdown / Dips Machine	Bench Dips / Band Triceps Extension
Quads	Barbell Back Squat	Dumbbell Goblet Squat	Leg Press Machine	Bodyweight Squats / Band Squats
Hamstrings	Barbell Romanian Deadlift	Dumbbell Stiff-Leg Deadlift	Seated / Lying Leg Curl Machine	Glute Bridge / Band Hamstring Curl
Glutes	Barbell Hip Thrust	Dumbbell Step-Ups	Glute Kickback Machine	Single-Leg Glute Bridge / Band Kickbacks
Calves	Barbell Standing Calf Raise	Dumbbell Seated Calf Raise	Calf Raise Machine	Bodyweight Calf Raises / Band Calf Raises
Abs / Core	Barbell Rollouts (Advanced)	Weighted Russian Twists	Cable Crunches	Planks / Hanging Leg Raises

The Pump

You've probably already experienced this, the tingling sensation in your muscles after certain exercises. This is the blood that runs to your muscles and is also called 'the pump'. It is a sign that your muscles have been working and your muscles swell considerably as a result, just measure your bicep with a tape measure before a workout and then after. This can easily vary an inch! Unfortunately, the pump decreases again after a while, but it is a nice indication of where your muscle wants to grow to. At some point, the pump from a few years ago suddenly has become your normal muscle size! Muscle growth takes time and energy, but if you stay consistent and eat enough and healthy, your muscles will grow.

The mind-muscle connection

Sometimes you don't feel the muscle you're training. This is often the case with hardgainers and usually with the bicep muscle. You can fix this. A simple way to do this is to look at the muscle you are training. So look at your bicep when you train it. Always do the movement slowly as previously prescribed. A whole movement, so complete the movement until your muscle is stretched out a little, and back again until you have real muscle contraction.

It seems like a bit of quackery, but this is really scientifically proven (https://pubmed.ncbi.nlm.nih.gov/26700744/). Bodybuilders have been using this technique for decades.

Finally

Don't stop if you don't see immediate muscle growth. For many of us hardgainers, it takes a while before it really becomes visible. Those first months I also grew fast, but then it stopped, at least in terms of visible growth. But I did get stronger and could lift more and more weight. I have kept track of everything from the beginning, just like I have recommended to you. I tracked all the repetitions and all the weights I did per exercise and muscle group. I started the chest press with dumbbells of 10 kilos each for 3 sets of 10 repetitions. Now I'm at 30kg per dumbbell for 3 sets of 10 reps. That is quite a nice growth and relatively heavy for my stature and weight. But as mentioned earlier, heavy lifting is secondary to time-under-tension and proper form. I always pay attention to these rules when I go heavier, because they should not be compromised. Then your muscles do not grow or hardly grow, and you have a greater chance of injuries.

In the end, it took me more than a year before I really started to develop muscle definition. Because of all the beautiful stories I read and heard, I had expected earlier results. But no. It's the long haul that wins. Perseverance, as already mentioned. But I was able to pull this off and so can you!

You now have the knowledge and the ingredients to achieve your goal. You don't need to know or do more than this. Don't be tempted by the fitness marketing. Stay consistent, keep training. Then, you'll definitely be successful.

I got your back! If you have questions or trouble with something, send me or my team an email at info@fitterisbeter.nl (yes, that is with one 't').

Literature used

1. FITTER IS BETER, AFVALLEN EN GESPIERD WORDEN MAAR DAN ECHT, Luc Molenaar (2022), Publisher: Boekscout, ISBN 9789464680980

2. GUIDELINES FOR GOOD NUTRITION 2015, Health Council of the Netherlands, 4 November 2015

3. ALCOHOL IS HARMFUL TO THE MUSCLES, Trimbos Institute, shown on www.alcoholinfo.nl

4. TRANSVET, Nutrition Center, displayed on www.voedingscentrum.nl/encyclopedie/transvet.asp xo

5. SUPERCOMPENSATION, Leiden University, shown on www.uscleiden.nl/nieuws/2014/06/23/supercompensatie/

6. WHAT ARE FAST-TWITCH MUSCLE FIBERS? Tiffany Ayuda, November 6, 2022, listed on: www.health.com/fitness/fast-twitch-muscle-fibers

7. HEALTHY EATING PYRAMID, Harvard T.H. Chan, School of Public Health, as published on: hsph.harvard.edu

About the Author

Luc Molenaar is a highly experienced coach and trainer specializing in helping hardgainers—those who struggle to build muscle no matter how hard they try. He's also the author of several bestselling books on muscle building, fitness, and nutrition.

Luc has coached people from all over the world, guiding them toward stronger, more muscular bodies through clear, science-based strategies. He's spoken at international seminars and draws from a deep background in muscle physiology, anatomy, training, and nutrition. His education includes studies at the University of Colorado Boulder and the Open University, among others.

But what really sets Luc apart? He's a hardgainer himself. He knows exactly what it's like to battle for every pound of muscle, to constantly eat yet stay lean, and to push through the frustration and stay motivated. That personal experience is what fuels his no-nonsense coaching approach — and makes him a go-to expert for people facing the same struggle.

Luc's writing style is direct, practical, and easy to follow. He doesn't sugarcoat the truth or waste time on hype. He gives you the tools that actually work. His books have sold worldwide, and this latest edition is already in its second print run.

If you're ready to finally make gains, you're in good hands.

www.ingramcontent.com/pod-product-compliance
Lightning Source LLC
Chambersburg PA
CBHW051821250726
48659CB00005B/1617